I0428698

Power Chairs
And
Electric Mobility
Scooters

Mema Manna

Copyright © 2010 Mema Manna

All rights reserved.

Table of Contents

Chapter 1

The Building Blocks For Outdoor Mobility Scooters and Power Chairs

Mobility scooters are designed to assist those who have difficulty with the tasks and opportunities associated with daily living.

They can be designed for indoor or outdoor use, with some models being middle of the road and designed to accommodate both indoor and outdoor use.

However, there are particular construction and user needs that have to be met in order for a mobility scooter to perform outdoors at optimum levels.

A good portion of what is necessary for mobility scooters to be more effective and comfortable for the rider outdoors lies within the construction and design of the base unit.

Base units are the bodies of mobility scooters and are often referred to as a platform or base plate.

Typically, base units consist of a frame constructed of aluminium steel or composite materials with a composite or fibreglass floor to support the seat, feet, battery and tiller, also known as the steering column.

Base units also include the mobility scooter's drive train.

The mobility scooter's manoeuvrability and its suitability for indoor or outdoor use in large part depends upon the characteristics of the base unit such as its turning radius, the size of its wheelbase, its ground clearance, and its overall dimensions.

It is important to evaluate the base for safety features, including its overall stability. A scooter should not tip easily during sharp turns or while climbing a curb.

Anti-tip wheels should be included as part of the frame to help support and stabilize the scooter.

Most rear wheel drive mobility scooters are intended to negotiate more rugged terrain and are usually equipped with rear anti-tips to support the scooter on hills.

The drive train is a critical part of the base unit and provides either front or rear wheel drive for the mobility scooter.

Front-wheel drive is usually found on smaller scooters designed primarily to be used indoors or outdoors on flat or paved surfaces.

The motor of the front wheel drive scooter is located over the front wheels and drives only those wheels.

Because of the motor and wheel configuration, front wheel drive mobility scooters usually do not have chains or belts and are powered by smaller motors.

The front wheels pull the weight of the rider and the scooter making them less capable of handling steep inclines, climbing curbs and managing rough terrain.

Rear wheel drive mobility scooters are powered by motors connected to the rear axle, either via a chain, a belt, a transaxle unit, or a combination of these components.

Because the mobility scooter is driven by the rear wheels, they push the combined weight of the unit and the rider, rather than pull it like the front wheel drive models.

The combined weight of the rider, the motor, and the batteries over the rear wheels, generally create better traction than that is usually provided by front-wheel drive models.

The increased traction combined with the more powerful motors used on rear-wheel drive scooters results in better climbing ability.

Rear-wheel-drive scooters also have a greater maximum speed, a longer travelling range between battery charges, and a larger rider weight capacity.

These mobility scooters have a wider wheel base and a greater overall length, making some models less manoeuvrable and unsuitable for indoor use.

Chapter 2

Mobility Scooters Make For Easy Travel

Mobility scooters make short distance travel easier for
someone in need of assistance. Independent travel and daily
life become a little easier and enjoyable for the elderly or
people with a condition that makes it difficult for them to
walk or who may tire easily when walking.

For people in need, this motorized scooter not only makes travel easy,
It decreases their reliance on others and promotes the continuation of
an independent lifestyle.

These people may be suffering from the typical symptoms that affect
the ability to walk due to the natural process of aging or from a variety
of conditions that can make walking challenging and uncomfortable
including Arthritis, Multiple Sclerosis and Muscular Dystrophy.

As long as the rider has some ability to walk a few steps and has
adequate upper body strength and dexterity to operate and control the
scooter, a mobility scooter can make all kinds of limited travel easy for
those once limited to wheelchairs or dependent upon others.

Although manual chairs or walkers also assist those who have difficulty
walking, they also put a lot of strain on the upper body, especially the
arms and shoulders.

Not only can this strain can be eliminated with a mobility scooter, but
the individual is much less likely to fall down from a scooter or
fall off the seat of the scooter.

Some of the activities those who use a mobility scooter may once again
enjoy, even with their afflictions, are exploring shopping malls,
department stores, and grocery stores.

By alleviating the physical exertion required to walk, a mobility scooter enables the rider to advance through stores and shops without tiring and with the ability to steer their own course. A nice walk down the main street of a village or down a walkway at the park with family and friends need not be missed with the help of a mobility scooter. Sometimes just getting around the house can be difficult, and a mobility scooter can be a valuable source of independence.

Those who have difficulty walking but still perform work from a desk at home will find that a mobility scooter serves well as a stationary seat that swivels from side to front to easily accommodate and transport the rider to and from desks, file cabinets and office equipment without absorbing the physical strength needed to walk.

In addition, mobility scooters make travel easy for themselves!

The majority of mobility scooters can be disassembled into a few component parts and be stowed easily in the trunk of a car.

This makes the mobility scooter especially helpful for outings with friends and family.

Breaking down the scooter is not difficult and quite manageable if approached by one or two people with average physical strength and agility.

Mobility scooters can be gasoline powered, but you will find the majority are powered by electricity.

Electric mobility scooters will either have one or two batteries.

These batteries sit on-board the base platform, which also supports the feet and the seat.

The batteries are charged with a standard charger using a standard electrical outlet, making recharging easy-and continued travel enjoyable!

Chapter 3

Go Mobile With An Electric Scooter

The world is getting smaller and smaller as the population grows. And with the increasing number of vehicles being manufactured every month just to meet the rising demand for transportation, buying a car with the expected magnitude of traffic jams seems like an impractical idea.

It is for this reason that a lot of us have turned to scooters, which are comparatively lightweight, easier to maintain, and a whole lot cheaper to buy and take care of.

And, more recently, thanks to the innovative mind, electric mobility scooters have been introduced to the market.

The main goal of an electric mobility scooter is to provide convenience. Because traffic can be such a headache, the size of scooters allows its riders to just breeze through and get to their destinations even faster than taking a car or a cab on a normal day.

Because scooters have varying speeds, thrill seekers (and people who are always on the go) will benefit greatly from this piece of equipment. An electric mobility scooter is a little expensive compared to the regular gas-powered scooter, but this is primarily because its popularity has not peaked yet.

In some countries, electric mobility scooters have not even been heard of, so it's not likely that it's price would go down anytime in the next few years.

However, as more and more people become aware of its existence, and its many advantages, it will definitely be more available and accessible over the long term.

The best use for an electric mobility scooter is for the handicapped and the elderly.

Because both have difficulty travelling from one location to another, electric mobility scooters will allow them to effortlessly move about. Senior citizens and handicapped persons will no longer feel like they're too dependent on their care givers because with an electric mobility scooter, they can already get to any place they want without having to ask for help.

The downside to an electric mobility scooter, however, is that it needs to be charged to work.

If there is no electricity, the scooter will be useless. However, some people still find that it beats having to deal with erratic gas price increases.

Over time, perhaps, more people will appreciate the electric scooter, especially if it is sold at a lower cost. But, until then, we hope that it catches on.

Chapter 4

Are Electric Scooters Also For Kids?

Among the portable and compact vehicles we have today, perhaps there is none the safer for kids than an electric scooter.

Of course, by kids, we mean those aged 10 and up, who already know better than to poke their fingers in places where they shouldn't.

So, to answer the question, yes, electric scooters can also be for kids' use.

The fact that electric scooters are very easy to use and do not require gas to run, kids do not find any problem handling it.

If the battery weakens, all they have to do is plug the unit to an electrical outlet and it already starts charging for the next use.

Compared to the gas powered scooter, an electric scooter is safer for kids' use because they don't have to keep revving the machine.

In addition, it doesn't emit harmful gases, so you don't have to worry about your kid getting sick.

But, what you do need to worry about is where your kid will likely go when he starts to get the hang of his electric scooter.

Primarily, electric scooters were made to provide convenience for people with limited mobility; that is, the elderly or the handicapped.

But even kids can use it also, as long as they are supervised by an adult.

The safest electric scooter model for kids is the four-wheeled scooter, because it is the most stable of all.

What is the about electric scooters that entices even kids? The fact that an electric scooter can get you someplace gives kids a semblance of adulthood, in that they get to travel in a piece of equipment even without the knowledge of how to drive a car.

An electric scooter is great to bring along during picnics or trips to the beach.

Your kids will surely enjoy driving it around and showing it off to their friends.

Finally, while electric scooters are relatively safe for kids' use, it should never be operated without adult assistance.

Scooters, though safer, are still machines, and kids might get curious and injure themselves.

In addition, electric scooters can also run fast.

If your kid has no daredevil tendencies, then you have nothing to worry about.

But if speed is something he enjoys, you might not want to leave him alone with a scooter.

Chapter 5

Electric Scooters For Girls

There are lots of electric scooter models in the market today.
And since they are primarily created for the convenience of those who
are either handicapped or too old to move around, surely anybody can
use this piece of equipment --yes, even little girls.
Electric scooter sizes vary, but some can go as light as 22
pounds.
Girls can easily manoeuvrer scooters like these without having to ask
for help.
Thus, if you worry about your child growing tired with walking to
school every day, you can have her use a mini electric scooter.
At least, it's more stylish than going on an ordinary bike.
Little girls will enjoy riding around in electric scooters
because it gives them a sense of independence and adulthood.
Of course, you should not allow your child to go too far without an
adult in tow.
But if it's just for simple neighbourhood trips, surely there's nothing
wrong with your little girl operating an electric scooter.
A good brand would be the Zip'r Mobility, whose heaviest
model is just 29 pounds. In addition, it has a small basket in
front for your little girl to place her things in, much like the
bike she uses to go to school in the past.
 And if you're concerned about her riding home on dark weather,
you can breathe easy because it's also equipped with huge headlights.
Another is the Guardian, which has only 22 pounds as its heaviest
model.

Not only that, it also has 5 different seat adjustments for greater convenience.
so the next time your little girl celebrates her birthday, why not gift her with a nice little electric scooter?
Not only is safe and functional, but they are also stylish enough to proudly show off to her friends.

Chapter 6

Mobility Scooters That Make It In The Fast Lane

Mobility scooters have made a tremendously positive impact on the ability of those with physical challenges to perform their daily activities and participate in social events.
Although mobility scooters are intended to be of physical assistance and are not manufactured or designed essentially for speed, many experienced riders already know and enjoy the benefits they receive from their mobility scooter, but they may wish they could move just a little bit quicker.
There are a few mobility scooters that are faster than others. Fast mobility scooters might be appreciated by those who use their scooter to run local errands or for those who visit parks, golf courses, playgrounds and other outdoor attractions where a good amount of territory is generally covered at a moderate pace throughout the course of the visit.
A fast mobility scooter will allow the user to keep up with friends and family and enjoy many of the same sites.
When we are considering fast as it relates to electric mobility scooters, it is important to note that electric mobility scooters range in power and speed from approximately 5 mph to about 13 mph. The faster models are generally intended for outdoor use as opposed to indoor use, where travelling speed is usually not a very high concern.
As a general guideline, rear wheel drive mobility scooters will tend to be faster than front wheel drive models. Front wheel drive models tend to have a less powerful motor

providing power to the front wheel or wheels which pull the rider and the scooter.

Whereas a rear wheel drive mobility scooter is driven by the rear wheels which push, as opposed to pull, the combined weight of the scooter and the rider.

This motor and wheel configuration also permits the use of a larger motor and therefore distributes more power.

Pride Mobility Products Corporation knows a little bit about speed. This fast growing company was founded in 1986 and has taken the fast track to over $76 million in annual sales! Their brand name is almost synonymous with mobility scooters.

Pride Mobility produces a wide variety of mobility scooters that can be used on just about any terrain. Amongst those who have purchased Pride's brand of mobility scooters are the elderly and disabled including well known celebrities like scientist Stephen Hawking and actor Verne Troyer of "Austin Powers" fame.

Pride Mobility offers a fast mobility scooter introduced as the Wrangler PMV.

For approximately $3500 you can be travelling at 10 mph.

The Wrangler is a rugged mobility scooter intended for outdoor use. Thirteen inch deep tread tires help to make the Wrangler reliable and fast even on the roughest terrain.

It uses two 100AH batteries and has two motors for ultimate traction. The seven inch ground clearance will help to ensure that you don't get stuck in a tough spot.

The rugged construction of the Pride Mobility Wrangler line of mobility scooters does not compromise the comfort and convenience that are incorporated into all of Pride's designs.

The Wrangler comes standard with a high back seat that is available in your choice of size and colour and with flip back arm rests and a head rest for comfort.

For those who still enjoy golfing but not the travel on the course, additional options available for the Wrangler include a golf bag holder that will turn your mobility scooter into the ultimate golf cart making the Wrangler a fast, convenient and personalized way to get to the 18th hole!

Chapter 7

All About Electric Scooters

We've heard about electronic scooters already, but don't really understand what it means. And while we ARE aware that electronic scooters run on, well, electricity, there's still more we need to know.

E-scooters function by linking a battery and a motor the adult kick scooter, which is found in standard gas powered scooters. Speeds and brakes are controlled via a switch that is attached to the handlebar.

And because electronic scooters are a fairly new invention, laws governing them are still in process, so, technically, no rules are in place.

While there are also gas powered scooters, electric motor scooters are more convenient to use. This is because you no longer need to go to the gas station to fill up. All you need to do is plug the electric motor scooter into an electrical outlet and wait a couple of hours for it recharge fully.

After which, you can start enjoying another trip around the neighbourhood again.

Electronic scooters have varying speeds, too. The slowest could be at just 10 miles per house, while others can go for as fast at 30 miles per hour, enough to be included in several racing events.

In addition, these are also some scooters that can easily go uphill and cut through headwinds.

E-scooters glide on the road so the feeling of literally cruising the block is there.

It's also very useful when you need to do quick errands and short trips to the grocery store.

And because it's a pretty new vehicle, it is also a good way to meet new people, as it makes a very interesting conversation piece.

Problems with traffic will also be a thing of the past as scooters can easily manoeuvrer through any tight jam.

Never again will you be late for an appointment.

Electric motor scooters also come in portable and foldable versions. If you travel around a lot, you can simply fold up or disassemble your electric motor scooter and the plane won't even scold you for it.

Electric scooters can go as light as 22 pounds.

You can also say goodbye to having to worry about gas money (though you might see your electric bill rise).

Scooters are also so compact that you are allowed to bring them on public transports like planes, buses and trains.

Gas powered scooters do not have this privilege. Not only that, you are not a contributor to global warming and noise as they do not emit fumes and are very silent workers.

Although most people buy e-scooters as 'toy", it is a lot functional than it's perceived.

In summary, electric scooters are fast becoming the transportation of choice by many people, not just hobbyists and those with limited mobility.

And because demand for this equipment is increasing, it is likely to become more accessible and affordable in the years to come.

Chapter 8

Can Electric Scooters Go Fast?

There is no doubt that an electric scooter can get you someplace, but the issue of how fast it can go is something that deserves discussion.

People often have this misconception that because electric scooters were designed primarily for the elderly and the handicapped, it cannot pick up speed.

This is where they are wrong.

While electric scooters are not as fast as gas powered scooters, they are not lacking in the speed department.

In fact, some electric scooter models can be as fast as a little over ten miles per hour.

So if you're thinking of organizing an electric scooter race, you won't be embarrassed.

Because the concept of an electric scooter is fairly new, not many people accept it as a real mode of transportation. Most of us are still stuck with the wheelchair concept so we don't really see electric scooters as anything more but an improved version of a wheelchair in a more chic and hip form.

It's about time to tell the world that electric scooters are more than what the majority perceives of them.

The speed of electric scooters and their overall performance should never be underestimated. Given the heavy traffic we are experiencing nowadays, which really are not showing signs of relenting anytime soon, we might find that owning an electric scooter and going to work with it is one of the most practical decisions we will ever make.

Electric scooters are not just for those with limited mobility. Even a perfectly healthy person can take advantage of an electric scooter.

In addition, the fact that electric scooters no longer need gas to go fast is comforting, especially at a time of skyrocketing oil and fuel prices. And while it does hike up our electricity bills, most people see that as a small price to pay for huge convenience electric scooters bring in.

Electric scooters are a very practical buy. In fact, they might even be more practical than buying a car. It doesn't protect you from the rain, though. But if you're looking to get somewhere fast, you can always rely on an electric scooter to serve its function.

Chapter 9

Comparing Gas Powered And Electric Scooters

Given the times we live in today, where purchase rate of consumer goods are continuing to rise and the price of oil and gas not planning to back down anytime soon, we definitely need an alternative means of transportation that is both efficient and environmentally friendly.

The invention and introduction of electric scooters has been a godsend to many individuals, who used to complain of always being late because of heavy traffic or of the unabating price of gas.

Electric scooters are fairly new so the demand is not up yet, but, over time, when the market catches on, it won't be a surprise if we make it our transportation of choice.

What is the difference between a gas powered and electricity powered scooter? Well, aside from the obvious, gas powered scooters are said to run faster, though this could arguable as some models of electric scooters are able to perform in speeds that rival regular scooters.

But, perhaps, the best thing about the coming of electric scooters is that its use does not contribute to the slow thinning of the ozone layer.

Gas scooters burn fuel to run, leaving some sort of chemical dust every time they are revved.

With an electric scooter, however, there's no smoke.

Those who criticize electric scooters say that while it does eliminate worry over gas prices, the electricity bill will then become a problem.

Electric scooters need to be charged before they can run.

So if you're a heavy user, you might find yourself recharging a couple of time or more every day.

However which way we see it, gas powered scooters and electric scooters each have their own pros and cons. If a bigger electricity bill is something you can live with, then getting an electric scooter is a good and practical decision. But if being environmentally friendly is not a very huge issue for you and you don't have enough funds to finance the rather expensive electric scooter, gas powered scooters will serve you well.

Chapter 10

An Introduction To Medical Mobility Scooters

A mobility scooter is similar to an electric scooter or motor scooter in function and construction. However, additional power wheelchair type features and options make mobility scooters an excellent form of transportation for anyone who has good arm strength and upper body balance but needs occasional assistance.

Elderly people, and those who have progressive conditions that challenge their ability to walk, appreciate and benefit from the aid and convenience of a mobility scooter.

Users of the mobility scooter can usually walk to some degree, But have greater difficulty with slopes and longer distances.

The first mobility scooter was built in 1968 by a Mr. Alan Thieme in Bridgeport, Michigan.

Mr. Thieme created this front wheel drive scooter to assist a family member with multiple sclerosis regain some of their independent mobility.

The basic components of today's mobility scooters are two rear wheels with a seat above them, a flat area upon which to put the feet that also holds the seat and power source, and a steering column with handlebars to steer either one or two front wheels.

There are gasoline powered mobility scooters, though the majority of those manufactured are electric.

The more popular electric mobility scooter runs with one or two batteries on-board the scooter.

If you need more power to overcome steep hills and slopes, you will be better served with two batteries which will deliver more power than one.

These batteries are charged with a standard charger that connects to a typical electrical outlet.

The steering column, located centrally at the front of the scooter, is referred to as the tiller.

The tiller controls forward, reverse and speed controls with finger controls, a thumb paddle or a switch.

Mobility scooters are available in front wheel drive or rear wheel drive.

In general, front wheel drive mobility scooters will accommodate a rider up to 250 lbs. and are more convenient for indoor use due to their smaller size. Rear wheel drive mobility scooters can be used indoors and outdoors and will accommodate a weight of up to 350 lbs. There are also heavy duty rear wheel drive mobility scooters, which differs from the regular rear wheel drive mobility scooters in that it can accommodate riders up to 500 lbs.

Because scooters usually have automatic braking, coasting is not an option.

You must use the finger, thumb or switch style controls to be in command of all movement.

You will need to press and release the controls gently to gradually increase and decrease speed.

There is usually a control that will allow you set the maximum speed for the scooter as well.

A mobility scooter will not be difficult to operate and control as long as you have adequate upper body strength and control and they can be broken down into parts quite easily making them convenient to pack into the trunk of a car for an outing with friends and family.

Anyone with systemic or disabling body conditions that is still able to stand and walk a few steps, control the steering tiller and sit in an upright position without torso support will appreciate the assistance of a mobility scooter and the sense of independence it can provide.

Chapter 11

How Can I Find Used Electric Mobility Scooters?

There are a number of different types of mobility scooters. Each has their own advantages and disadvantages, which can be looked at objectively by individual parties and those who are interested in purchasing the items.

However, they often can be very expensive.

Most people that have looked into purchasing these types of items have noticed that they can be quite an investment. While there are some situations in which an individual's insurance company will either pay for or help the individual pay for such an apparatus, there are many people that are required to pay for the item on their own if they wish to use one or feel like they are needing such an item in their home in order to help them get around and go from one place to another with a sense of ease and convenience.

Because of the cost, many people will actually be able to benefit from purchasing used electric mobility scooters. These are scooters, powered by electricity which is typically charged for a period of time before the scooter is used to transport the owner, that have been handled before by previous owners.

They are discounted in price because they have been used. In most cases, these scooters are still in very good condition and will meet all the requirements that the individual has as

http://www.electricmobilitychairs.com

for why they need such a device, but the used electric mobility scooters will actually cost much less for the individual.
Not unlike the degradation in the value of
cars, a used scooter is simply cheaper than a new scooter,
and the reason for this is typically not because the scooter
works any less effectively than the new model works.
Upon learning this, many people become more interested in the models of used electric mobility scooters that they can purchase, but they may not readily know where they can go in order to purchase one.
After all, these devices are seen in public quite often but there are very few scooter stores to which an individual can go and make their purchase.
Instead, individuals need to be a little more creative when it comes to trying to find such items.
First, there is the internet. Many people are able to utilize this resource and find a used scooter that they can purchase and have shipped to them.
While the internet is a great resource, this is not the only way in which a person can purchase such an item.
Instead, they can also look through newspaper classified ads or even place a classified ad informing other readers that they are looking for such an item.
If a reader has a scooter that they are willing to sell,
they can contact the individual and set up the exchange.
Without reading the ad, individuals may have not been thinking about selling the items, but upon reading the ad and knowing that there is a specific need for their item they may be more willing to part with their used electric mobility scooters if they are not longer needed and being used.

Chapter 12

How To Choose Used Electric Scooters

Electric scooters are a relatively new concept, so the demand for them right now is just staring to grow. Thus, it is not surprising that it's price remains at $600 to $900 levels. While this can be a put off for many potential buyers, the fact That you can also buy used versions of these electric scooters is a comforting thought.

Buying a used electric scooter is a practical decision. Most of the used electric scooters being resold were previously owned by people who just receive the units from Medicare, so finding a reasonable price for them is not difficult. You can scan the Internet, local Classifieds, and garage sales for sales like these.

There are many Internet Web sites that offer used electric scooters. The benefit of this is that you are most likely to find exactly what you are looking for online, as opposed to visiting physical sales, which have limited choices.

If shopping online intimidates you, be sure to transact only with secure sites to be on the safe side.

Of course, as with any purchase, check the scooter for any signs of damage or overuse before you buy it. Find out where the scooter came from and how it was used.

At this point, you will have to act on good faith, as you really can't be sure if the seller is telling you the truth.

But, hey, if you're getting it rock-bottom cheap, it's a risk you will need to take.

The things you will need to look at when you're buying used scooter is its mileage, years of use, and past repairs. If the unit still covered by a warranty, you're lucky. But more often than not, these units have been resold because they have gone past the warranty stage.

When it comes to owning your own electric scooter, there is no need to go all out with the expense. With a little ingenuity, you can find the perfect electric scooter at more than half the cost. Just be patient enough to look for it.

Chapter 13

What Are Standing Mobility Scooters?

By looking at the phrase mobility scooters, many people are able to conclude that the device is an apparatus which is able to move the individual from one location to another, with limited, if any, strain and stress on the body of the individual. Upon consideration, many people may then go on to realize that they have been able to observe these apparatuses in their everyday life, even if they did not realize it at the time.

There are many stores that will offer mobility scooters with baskets attached in order to make shopping at the store easier for individuals that would need that type of support and help. However, the new phrase that is standing mobility scooters may cause some individuals to pause and reflect on what this could be.

The words standing and mobility would initially seem to contradict themselves, which could be confusing for someone to come to terms with when they are trying to come up with an acceptable conclusion as to what this device could be. In the end, however, individuals will understand that the words do not contradict each other, but rather that each of the terms refers to something more specific about the scooter in general, and that they in fact merely go on to help describe the scooter in more detail.

The attention to detail helps individuals to more accurately and easily locate and research the types of scooters that would be most applicable to them and their situation.

While some mobility scooters will move the individual from one place to another while they are seated on the scooter, standing mobility scooters provide the same function, but with the individual in a different position.

Instead of sitting, these scooters allow the individual to stand up on them and be transported in this manner and fashion.

There are actually many reasons as to why this type of scooter may be considered to be more attractive to the individual as opposed to the different types of mobility scooters that can be provided to individuals.

Some people do not need to be seated which they move about. For example, an individual with one broken foot may be able to benefit from using a mobility scooter, but these can be expensive and help the individual to put on some weight as a result of not being as active.

Instead, a standing mobility scooter may be used, enabling the individual to stand up and be more comfortable, but still move around much faster than if they had been on crutches.

In most cases, they are also much less expensive since they are smaller.

In contrast, an individual with two broken feet would not be able to use a standing mobility scooter, simply because then they would have to put pressure on their feet which cannot safely be done when the bones in the feet are broken.

The individual with two broken feet would then be limited to the mobility scooter that allows them to sit down on the scooter and still be moved from one location to another location.

Chapter 14

Tips On Using Electric Scooters

Electric scooters are easy to use and manoeuvrer, but any machine, when not properly operated can result in injury. Thus, even if you somehow underestimate the potential of an electric scooter to cause accidents, it is still very much possible, especially if you don't know how to ride it.

Here are some safety tips you should consider when purchasing and operating electric scooters.

- Buy a scooter that's right for your size. If you're too big for the unit, the chances of it's toppling over, forward or backward is huge.

On the contrary, if you're too small, you might have a lot trouble making it go your way.

- Be careful with the installation process. There are some electric scooters where you will still have to do some preliminary work for it to be perfectly functional. If you doubt your ability to follow instructions, have it done at the store where you purchased it before you bring it.

If it is a pride issue, think of it this way: suppose you forced yourself to install those parts yourself and they fell apart, who's to blame?

- Buy an electric scooter that fits your lifestyle. If you're the type who likes to go camping, don't buy a scooter that's too light or feeble to use on slightly rough roads. A four-wheel electric scooter is perfect for this kind of activity.

A two wheeler could prove too light for comfort.

- Make sure all the features are working before you head out.

Don't be too confident that having a broken headlight is okay. You never know, you could get stuck somewhere and be left riding in the dark.

Overall, the point of proper electric scooter use is maximizing functionality. IF you have no need for a four wheeler, don't get it. It will only take up space in your garage.

Buy only what you need to spare yourself from the hassle of having to lug the thing around when one of its parts conks out.

In addition to that is safety. No electric scooter is a good scooter if you don't know how to use it well. Instead of getting convenience, you might only subject yourself to injury.

Chapter 15

Form, Function And Style With Pride Mobility Scooters

Pride Mobility Products Corporation is the manufacturer of the number one selling brand of mobility scooters in the United States. Putting a tremendous amount of effort into designing and manufacturing high quality mobility scooters is just one of the reasons Pride Mobility has risen above the competition.

Their innovative designs and durable product lines help individuals who have difficulty walking participate in activities and events they might otherwise have to avoid.

A Pride Mobility Scooter helps an individual who is having some trouble getting around on their own to easily move themselves around the house, shopping mall, or village streets while allowing them to maintain their independence.

Pride Mobility Scooters are well respected in their industry for being more than just a means of transportation. Their scooters are designed with the reliability needs, comfort and convenience of the user being highly accounted for in their designs.

Pride Mobility Scooters are carefully constructed to be smooth riding, quiet and easy to operate.

The individual is never forgotten during the design of a Pride Mobility Scooter and personal style and taste preferences are also taken into consideration during the design process. A large selection of models that accommodate different individual needs and budgets are available in a wide array of colours.

Convenient features and accessories help to ensure the rider
is able to move about with the least amount of physical exertion
and at a more than adequate level of personal comfort.
Pride Mobility Products Corporation has several authorized
sales and distribution centres throughout the United States.
These distributors represent the world leader in mobility
equipment and represent the Pride Mobility Scooter product
line and also provide service when necessary.
These authorized distributors are knowledgeable and experienced
at answering questions and making recommendations that
will help you select the Pride Mobility Scooter that is best for
the individual.
Some distributors will even allow a potential buyer to take
the mobility scooter out for on-site trials for a specific period of time.
A trial period allows the individual to more accurately determine
the scooters performance, and whether the controls, seating,
and leg room are sufficiently comfortable for long-term use.
The combination of style, solid performance and exceptional
value found with Pride Mobility Scooters is consistent
throughout their various models.
For many people who have conditions that adversely affect
their mobility, a Pride Mobility Scooter can be a cost effective
and attractive alternative to a motorized wheel chair.
For some a more attractive, less 'medical" appearance is an
important factor.
For others, greater flexibility is a primary consideration. For
those not requiring the sophisticated electronics or seating
systems of a powered wheelchair, the smaller price tag is
attractive.
Whatever the reason for considering a scooter, models should
be carefully evaluated for their capability to accommodate a
person's disability and meet the requirements of the intended use.
In addition to gathering information from a Pride Mobility
Scooter distributor, those who are purchasing their first Pride
Mobility Scooter should consult with their physician, therapist,
or other rehabilitation professional to determine whether a
mobility scooter is the best option and what functional features
are required to suit their individual needs.

Chapter 16

Reliable Mobility Scooters Begin At The Bottom

If you are on a limited budget in the market for a mobility scooter, you may want to dedicate a little bit of time to comparing prices. Mobility scooters are available from many different manufacturers and in various styles. Just a few of the features and options you will find enhancing [Peterborough Ont.] mobility scooters are specialty base plates or platforms, wheels or tires, and seats.

The options and features that differentiate one mobility scooter from the next should be selected according to your particular needs and intended usage.

The base plate, or platform, supports your feet, the seat, the tiller, or steering column, and the battery. The base plate determines the comfort and safety of the user and whether or not the scooter is designed for indoor or outdoor use.

The frames and support platforms of the base plates on [Peterborough Ont.] mobility scooters are typically constructed of steel, aluminium or composite materials. Mobility scooter base plates are customized by manufacturers and then identified by different model and style names presented to the consumer.

A mobility scooter intended for indoor use only will typically have a composite base plate to which adjustments have been made to the minimize the size of the wheelbase and amount of ground clearance as well as more precise manoeuvrability features to better accommodate the size and floor plan associated with a typical home.

Some models of [Peterborough Ont.] mobility scooters have

a longer length or an extendable base that can accommodate longer legs.

An increased base length will increase the turning cycle of the scooter; however a well constructed mobility scooter will not tip easily during sharp turns or inclines and will provide a smooth, stable ride. The size of the wheels on a mobility scooter determines the ability of the scooter to surmount obstacles and affects its stability. Mobility scooters usually have six, eight or ten inch wheels, and these are usually of equal diameter in the front and the back. Smaller wheels are generally found on front wheel drive mobility scooters intended for indoor use.

The larger the wheels, the more stable the ride and the larger and wider the tires the greater the ability of the mobility scooter to manage climbing curbs and maneuver over rough terrain. [Peterborough Ont.] Mobility scooters are available with either three or four wheels. Four wheeled mobility scooters tend to be more stable than those with three wheels, especially for curb climbing and turning sharp corners.

Three wheeled scooters have a smaller turning circle and tend to be easier to maneuver.

The most common types of tires are solid, pneumatic, puncture proof and deep tread tires.

Solid tires do not puncture or ever need inflating.

Pneumatic tires need to be inflated regularly to maintain air pressure and checked frequently as they can puncture. They do provide a more comfortable and smooth ride than solid rubber tires and punctures can be repaired with a relatively simple at home repair kit or by a local cycle shop or mobility scooter repair center.

Puncture proof tires are a compromise between solid and pneumatic tires.

They are made of an open cell rubber compound to help with the shock absorption.

Deep tread tires are available with different levels of tread. The deeper the tread, the greater the ability of the mobility scooter to provide increased grip and stability on curbs as well as on slopes, muddy grass and rough or uneven ground.

Chapter 17

Mobility Scooters And Peterbough Ont.

All over the world, there are many people that are looking for mobility scooters. There are many reasons as to why individuals would want to use mobility scooters, and there are just as many places from which an individual could obtain a mobility scooter.

Ontario is just one of the many places in the world from which a person would want to be able to locate and utilize a scooter that offers mobility to the individual.

Peterborough, Ontario is one specific location in which individuals have been able to come to the conclusion that they would be able to benefit from a mobility scooter.

Scooters that offer mobility to the individuals that need it are advantageous for a number of different reasons. First of all, they allow individuals that would otherwise not be able to move about and interact with others to do so.

This can have a number of different types of effects on the individual, not the least of which would be increased motivation, social skills and convenience.

From that point on, these different benefits can go on, like a chain reaction, to benefit other areas of the individual's life as well.

Nonetheless, there are other advantages as well. For example, being able to move around with ease will help a person to stay motivated to continue doing things.

This is because there will not be the added stress and strain of

pressure, pain, or inconvenience when it comes to doing things.
Instead, the individual can focus on how convenient and effortless it is to move around and get things done with their mobility scooter, as opposed to trying to get these things done without the mobility scooters.
It will also allow the individual to get out and interact with others.
These alone can lift a person's spirits.
When an individual feels better and feels more confident, they are much more likely to stay positive and get better faster, if they are in a position that requires them to heal.
Studies have shown that the power of positive thinking has a number of benefits, and through mobility scooters many people are able to access these specific feelings.
They are potentially then able to help the individual heal faster simply because of the many positive effects that they can and may be able to provide for the individual that is using the scooter.
Even in Peterborough ont. Scooters mobility can be utilized in order to help residence get around.
They can purchase new or used scooters.
While there is not a huge difference between used scooters and new scooters, this will need to be determined on an individual basis since only the individual that would be using the mobility scooter could be able to correctly identify how they need their scooter to be.
Most used scooters that are being resold are in good condition, will be considered to be good running order and will have little damage to them.
In addition, they are often much cheaper.
The new scooters, however, often will come with a warrantee.
In the end, this decision needs to be left up to the individual investigating Peterborough ont. Scooters mobility.

Chapter 18

Yes, You Can Own A Pink Electric Scooter

Because an electric scooter is just like any other vehicle whose looks and design you can experiment with, nobody can tell you that a pink electric scooter is not possible.
In fact, if you want an electric scooter that's pink on one side and blue on the other, there really is nobody who can tell you it's not okay.
You are the master of your vehicle and surely you can do anything you want with it, even place a vinyl decal of your own face, if you wish.
But there is something about a pink electric scooter that is very appealing, especially if the owner is a girl or a child.
Guys are not spared from pink electric scooters, though, and have every right to own one.
Hey, it's a free country, right?
Just because you own a pink electric scooter doesn't mean you're on the fruity side.
Some electric scooter manufacturers already produce pink electric scooters for their various models.
 But if your particular unit does not come in that shade, you can always have it customized, just like any other vehicle.
You can either do it yourself using vinyl decals or an airbrush, or you can have it professionally done by somebody who also paints cars. Turning an electric scooter pink is the same as turning a car pink, so it's really not a hassle.
Since pink is not really a colour of choice for most people,

some electric scooter makers offer pink models as a limited edition version.

So if you want a factory original, you should watch out for these kinds of offers.

Besides, electric scooters are designed not just to be functional, but also stylish, so finding a pink electric scooter might not be a problem.

How choose to design your electric scooter is up to you.

Since you're the one who will be going around town in it, it would be nice to add a little, or a big, something to identify the vehicle as yours.

In addition, painting your electric scooter pink is a great deterrent for would-be thieves, who might have second thoughts trying to steal a vehicle that is very noticeable on the road.

Chapter 19

Frequently Asked Questions About Electronic Scooters

Here are some of the most frequently asked questions about electronic scooters, to give you a better understanding about its mechanism and why it is fast becoming popular these days.

How do electronic scooters work?

E-scooters function by linking a battery and a motor the adult kick scooter, which is found in standard gas powered scooters. Speeds and brakes are controlled via a switch that is attached to the handlebar.

And because electronic scooters are a fairly new invention, laws governing them are still in process, so, technically, no rules are in place.

Electronic scooters have varying speeds, too. The slowest could be at just 10 miles per house, while others can go for as fast at 30 miles per hour, enough to be included in several racing events. In addition, these are also some scooters that can easily go uphill and cut through headwinds.

Why are electric scooters so popular and why do people use them?

E-scooters glide on the road so the feeling of literally cruising the block is there. It's also very useful when you need to do quick errands and short trips to the grocery store. And because it's a pretty new vehicle, it is also a good way to meet new people, as it makes a very interesting conversation piece.

Problems with traffic will also be a thing of the past as scooters can easily maneuver through any tight jam. Never again will you be late for an appointment. Also, you can also say goodbye to having to worry about gas money (though you might see your electric bill rise).

What are the other advantages of electric scooters?

E-scooters are so compact that you are allowed to bring them on public transports like planes, buses and trains.

Gas powered scooters do not have this privilege.

Also, you are not a contributor to global warming and noise as they do not emit fumes and are very silent workers.

And though most people buy e-scooters as 'toy", it is a lot functional than it's perceived.

There are many other things you need to know about scooters, but the above information is generally what people ask about this amazing invention.

Apart from being a convenient mode of transportation and interesting toy, scooters can also be helpful to people with limited mobility, like the handicapped and senior citizens.

Indeed, the birth of electronic scooters has brought in so many benefits that a one page list won't suffice.

Chapter 20

Where To Find Service And Parts List For Pride Mobility Scooters

Pride Mobility Products Corporation is the privately owned company that manufacturers a very popular and respected line of mobility scooters.

This very successful company was founded in 1986 and has consistently grown, now exceeding $76 million dollars in annual sales.

It is obvious that many people are purchasing Pride Mobility's line of mobility scooters and for good reason – they are available in a wide variety of models and styles, moderately priced, features and durable.

But even the most reliable motor scooters need routine maintenance and care in order to operate at optimum levels at all times.

So, if you own a Pride Mobility scooter and want to keep it in optimum operating conditions, you will need to have a list of the parts applicable to your particular model mobility scooter and a reliable source from which to obtain Pride Mobility replacement parts, a price list, and, if necessary, access to an authorized service technician.

The operator's manual for a Pride Mobility scooter is provided at the time of purchase and includes a list of parts specific to the model purchased.

If by chance this manual has been lost, you can download a copy from Pride Mobility's website at www.pridemobility.com/resourcecenter .

The manual also supplies information on routine maintenance procedures, parts lists, repair options and troubleshooting advice.

The web site also provides a lot of useful information including their contact information so you can contact them directly for information regarding parts lists and repairs. Most distributors of Pride mobility scooters carry many of the consumable parts most often purchased such as batteries, tires and chargers.

Many carry convenient accessories such as cane or walking stick holders, oxygen holders, cup holders, baskets and canopies. However, should you been in need of a mechanical repair you will need to know where to obtain the appropriate replacement parts and possibly some help from an authorized service center.

Pride Mobility has authorized sales and service distribution arms throughout the United States.

Each authorized service center has parts lists for all Pride Mobility scooter models.

Should you be mechanically inclined and have already identified the parts you need, contacting one of Pride Mobility's authorized sales and service centers should be all you need to do to purchase the parts you need to do.

These authorized service centers also have technicians that have completed the required Pride Mobility repair training program to efficiently repair your mobility scooter with genuine high quality Pride Mobility parts.

Drop off and repair service is usually available should a Distribution center be within a short distance for you, and even house calls within a limited local area are an option from some providers.

Spinlife.com, LLC, is an authorized Pride Mobility sales and service distributor.

Their expert technical staff is well qualified to repair your mobility scooter using genuine parts from the manufacturer's recommendation list.

They also commit to finding someone who can help you with parts and repairs should they be unable to do so themselves. You can find out more about Pride Mobility Scooters and Spinlife.com LLC at:www.Spinlife.com

Chapter 21

The Advantage Of An Electric Scooter Over A Wheelchair

Wheelchairs have evolved over time to give greater comfort and convenience to people who have limited mobility. From simple manual operations, wheelchairs can now be operated automatically with just a few clicks of the button, allowing its riders to perform daily mundane tasks a lot easier and faster. However, the geniuses that made automatic wheelchairs have also come up with a new invention that is expected to trump wheelchairs in the years to come -- electric scooters. Not only are electric scooters easier to use and operate compared to wheelchairs but they are also more chic and stylish that it's not really embarrassing to go around town in it. Perhaps the biggest advantage of owning an electric scooter is that it takes you to places farther than the wheelchair can. A wheelchair is okay to use if you're just inside the house or in a small enclosed area.

But if you want to go to the grocery store or the nearby park, an electric scooter is your ally.

While it does not go as fast as gas powered scooters, it is fast nevertheless and can even travel for several miles before needing another recharge.

In addition, with electric scooters, all you have to do is plug it in to store power. Its battery life lasts depending on its usage, but, still, it remains better by several points over wheelchairs.

The good news is, with the growing demand for electric

scooters, prices are also starting to go down. You can buy an electric scooter for as low as $580, and can even get one for a cheaper price if you scour auctions, sales, and used electric scooter offers.

Of course, whenever you purchase something, check it first for signs of damage and find out where it has been before you make any decision.

The convenience afforded by an electric scooter is something an ordinary wheelchair cannot parallel.

Even automatic wheelchairs still cannot hold a candle to electric scooters.

Chapter 22

CTM Mobility Scooters

If an individual is looking for a scooter that is made by a company that is reliable and dependable, then they may need to look no further than CTM mobility scooters.

The models that they are able to produce can be purchased by the general public at large.

The company understands that individuals need different things. One person will need such a device for the rest of their life, while another person may just need it for a few months.

There are so many different people with specific needs, and if a company does not offer different models when it comes to their mobility scooters, they will not be able to appeal to as many consumers as they would otherwise have been able to do.

As a result, companies such as CTM have been able to come up with different designs and different models to offer their customers. However, this does not stay limited to the way that the CTM mobility scooters are able to look and appear. Rather, they are also different when it comes to the motors that are offered and the power source of the individual CTM mobility scooters.

For those who do not need them, these things may seem like simple and trivial aspects of such devices that do not really matter in the long run.

But to those that are familiar with the CTM mobility

scooters and who do need one in order to get around and be transported from one place to another, the knowledge that these different aspects are very important and useful when it comes to making a decision as to which type of scooter would best suit their immediate needs as well as their financial planning procedures.

There are two different types of power sources when it comes to mobility scooters, and the type that is best for the individual will vary from person to person, since different things are convenient to different people.

Batteries will run some of the mobility scooters, while others will need to be charged for a period of time before they are used. In cases that rely on the power source as an important and vital piece to the decision making process, individuals that do not have the time to keep their mobility scooter charged, individuals that are constantly on the go, would likely be better off with a battery that can be replaced as opposed to one that needs to be charged every so often.

There are also differences when it comes to the motors of the scooters. Some people will be much more demanding of their scooters as opposed to others.

Just for example, if a person is using their scooter all the time and they have a lot of hills on their property, they will likely need a more powerful motor in their scooter in order to keep them effective.

By contrast, if a person is going to be moving on flat surfaces for the most part and they will not be very demanding on their scooter, they would be just as happy with a mobility scooter that does not use such a strong motor, since it would effective be a waste of money if they never need to use its extra capabilities in motor form.

Chapter 23

Cheap Electric Scooters

Electric scooters are the 'in' thing for those with limited mobility nowadays. Senior citizens and the handicapped find that using an electric scooter is more convenient that getting around in a wheelchair because aside from the fact that they are easier to operate, they can also get them farther. Wheelchairs can go only as far as a few meters, but scooters can run for several miles.

But since electric scooters are still a relatively new concept, the price tag can be a bit overwhelming. For an ordinary electric scooter, you stand to spend around $700. This can be pretty steep for someone who works within a fixed budget. However, this doesn't mean that it is only for the rich. You can actually buy cheap electric scooters, if you only know how and where to find them.

First off, the Internet is a haven for just about any kind and brand of cheap electric scooter. You can buy an electric scooter for a lower price because it is out of date or if it has already been used. Before you make your purchase, however, you should find out the unit's history first and if it had undergone repairs in the past. Also, check its mileage and any signs of wear.

Second, check out vehicle auctions. Some people trade in their electric scooters to get a loan with creditors, and if these people are not able to pay, their scooters are sold to the public at a very low price.

Not all vehicle auctions have electric scooters in their roster, but it's definitely worth a try.

Third, watch out for store sales. Yes, even electric scooters are included in motor parts sales, sometimes, so it's best to be friends with the staff so you get information about a sale earlier than anybody else does.

This way, you get a head start on the kinds of electric scooters available and you can search the Internet for reviews.

Cheap electric scooters are possible, so if you don't have much money, you don't have to worry.

All you need is a little bit of skill, ingenuity and resourcefulness to catch the sales when they happen.

Chapter 24

Finding Mobility Scooters At A Discount

Mobility scooters can be of great assistance to anyone who has difficulty walking, but still has adequate upper body strength.

People can have difficulty walking for many reasons including arthritis, multiple sclerosis, muscular dystrophy and age related conditions.

People with these conditions are often on a limited budget and have many health related expenses.

So, a mobility scooter is often considered a luxury that simply cannot be afforded.

However, there are a variety of ways to purchase a mobility scooter at a discount price that will allow the rider to enjoy the physical and emotional benefits of a scooter without spending a fortune.

Mobility scooters alleviate the stresses that a manual chair or walker put on the upper body, as well as enable the rider to enjoy many activities that they might not otherwise have been able to participate in.

Although the rider of a mobility scooter must have enough strength and dexterity in the upper body to operate and manage the steering and hand operated controls of a mobility scooter, they need not have the additional strength and coordination required to operate a manual chair or walker.

This makes mobility scooters a viable and beneficial alternative for someone whose only other options might have been to refrain from activity or to purchase a more costly motorized wheel chair.

Mobility scooters are available worldwide at medical supply stores, specialty shops and from a multitude of online distributors. Your chances of getting a greater discount will most likely come from online distributors.

Shopping for a mobility scooter at a discount site online will enable you to research the various makes and models and comparison shop between distributor sites at your leisure. This will help you determine which make and model will suit your needs and also help to ensure you obtain the lowest discount price available.

There are several discount mobility scooter recommended websites where you will find terrific discount pricing as well as excellent customer service focused policies and procedures.

One of those sites is operated by Spinlife.com, LLC at www.spinlife.com , which allows us to browse through the many mobility scooters they have available at a discount.

With a variety of makes and models and limited or full featured versions, Spinlife.com certainly offers a great selection to choose from and discounts range up to 50% off list price - but that's not all. They have what they refer to as a 110% lowest price guarantee.

This guarantee means that if they verify that you found the identical item online at a lower price, they will discount their price by 110% of the price difference – talk about a great discount! Spinlife.com also provides helpful insurance eligibility information, free shipping and a fair and flexible return policy.

Another way to purchase a mobility scooter at a deep discount is to buy a second-hand or used mobility scooter. If you are willing to do without the most recent model, the newly enhanced features and the manufacturer's warranty associated with a brand new mobility scooter, you may be able to locate a good quality mobility scooter locally or on E Bay.

Chapter 25

Finding Cheap And Reliable Mobility Scooters

Many people who have difficulty walking take advantage of the generous availability of mobility scooters that are made available for use at several public facilities such as amusement parks, grocery stores and department stores. They can keep up with friends and family without overexerting themselves or go in their own direction without assistance from another individual.

Many of these people do not possess a personal mobility scooter of their own because they have a limited budget, although they would appreciate and gain so much from the physical assistance and the psychological benefits associated with maintaining their independence.

A cheap mobility scooter may be the affordable bridge that helps an individual cross over from a walk restricted lifestyle to a self-assisted and more independent lifestyle.

The mobility scooters available for use at public facilities are generally four wheeled and built for durability more than comfort and convenience.

Although comfort and convenience are typically adequately provided for, reliability and durability are the most important characteristics of any type of equipment that is made available for public use.

These mobility scooters are not cheap and would most likely be an over exaggerated version of a three or four wheeled model that would be more appropriate for a personal ownership.

A little bit of online research on the topic of medical mobility scooters should help you become more familiar with the different makes, models, features, advantages and limitations of mobility scooters.

As a general guideline, brand new mobility scooters range from just under $500 to well over $3000.

A mobility scooter with tons of options and features and a more powerful motor is not going to be one of the cheap models. In addition to particular specifications that may be provided, a clue as to the power of the motor is the number of batteries the mobility scooter has. A model that has two onboard batteries is likely to have a more powerful motor.

The more powerful motor makes conquering hills and steep slopes quicker and easier. A smaller motor will still conquer those hills but you just have to be a little more patient if you want to ride cheap. Trading a little time may still be better than being physically limited and assisted by others or not participating in an activity.

A walker is a relatively cheap piece of equipment that is designed to assist those who have trouble walking. Although effective at accomplishing their purpose, the individual using a walker must have a good amount of upper body strength and dexterity and enough energy and lung capacity to maneuver with a walker.

If the individual is this fortunate, they will be over utilizing these healthy body conditions to compensate for their inability to use their affected limbs.

A mobility scooter does require that the individual have an adequate amount of upper body strength in order to operate and manage the steering column and hand operated controls. However, the amount of strength and effort necessary is minimal with a cheap mobility scooter in comparison to a walker. A manual wheel chair presents some of the same disadvantages as a walker.

A motorized wheel chair is another option for those who have difficulty walking and they do not require the individual to have much upper body strength. However, they are not cheap and some find them to be too large and cumbersome for everyday activities in many places.

If you take the time to investigate the various mobility scooters available you may find a cheap yet valuable solution to a challenging physical and emotional problem.

Chapter 26

Electric Mobility Scooters Present A Viable Solution

To Physical Challenges

Electric mobility scooters can provide the elderly, disabled, and seriously ill freedom of movement. Mobility is a critical to just about every aspect of everyday living. Having some freedom of movement enhances a person's capability to learn, earn a living and interact with friends, family and community.

A large percentage of people with mobility limitations have permanent disabilities. Many people suffer from conditions that make walking an extremely difficult and painful task including arthritis, muscular dystrophy and multiple sclerosis.

These individuals benefit from a variety of mobility aids and devices to assist them in lead fulfilling and active lives.

The most popular forms of independently operated mobility equipment are electric mobility scooters and motorized wheelchairs. A motorized wheelchair is a form of personal transportation that typically has six wheels and is steered using a "joystick"type control mechanism.

Other names for the motorized wheelchair include, electric chair, power wheelchair and power chair.

A motorized wheelchair is usually equipped with outstanding manoeuvrability features that make them perfect for use in the home and will generally fit just about anywhere.

Power Chairs And Electric Mobility Scooters

Motorized wheelchairs are typically for in-door use.
The power mobility provided by electric wheelchairs has
made a dramatic difference in many people's lives.
The development of new technology in the industry has made it
possible for people to obtain smaller, more lightweight and
manoeuvrable motorized wheelchairs for use inside the
home allowing people to move about in small places and
complete their activities of daily living without being bedridden
or sent to nursing homes.
In comparison, electric mobility scooters have either three or
four wheels and steer much like a bicycle, using a set of handlebars
and hand operated control mechanisms. Electric mobility scooters
are ideal for indoor and outdoor activities, as they glide smoothly and
easily over a variety of surfaces. There are even portable electric
mobility scooters that will fit easily in the trunk of a car. Electric
mobility scooters are reliable, easy to operate, comfortable, safe and do
not have the more obvious medical appearance of a motorized
wheelchair. Today's electric mobility scooters have three or four wheels,
a steering column-known as a tiller-with handlebars and hand operated
control mechanisms and a platform that supports the seat, battery and
the riders feet.
Electric mobility scooters are much less physically strenuous than a
walker or manual wheelchair.
Although the rider of a mobility scooter must be physically able to
walk a few steps and have adequate upper body strength and dexterity,
they do not require the more substantial amount of strength and
dexterity necessary to operate a walker or manual wheelchair.
The swivelling captain's style seat of an electric mobility
scooter is typically easier than moving the foot
supports of a manual or motorized wheelchair.
In addition, electric mobility scooters are simple to maintain
and easily recharged using a standard electrical outlet and charger.
Physical impairments need not prevent someone from
participating in daily activities as well as special occasions
with family and friends.
Electric mobility scooters restore independence and freedom
of mobility to help promote an active lifestyle.

Chapter 27

A Guide To Buying An Electric Scooter

Scooters are the transportations of choice for a growing number of people in the world today. Because these vehicles are easy to manage and can manoeuvrer its way through just about any kind of traffic jam, more people are finding that it is practical compared to owning a car.

In fact, sales of scooters are increasing along with the worsening of traffic conditions, much to the delight of motor manufacturers. However, it doesn't end.

Scooter manufacturers have also thought of a way to make travelling a lot easier and convenient for people who are handicapped and senior citizens through the creation and introduction of the electric scooter.

As it name suggests, an electric scooter runs on electricity. It has to first be plugged into an outlet and charged before it can serve its purpose.

Are you looking to buy an electric scooter for your grandfather? There are many things you have to consider. And since buying electric scooters can be as confusing buying regular scooters (because there's so many kinds to choose from), it would be best to search what you need from the Internet to avoid wasting time at the showroom.

What are the things you need to consider when you buy an electric scooter? First, is it portable? Since you're buying for your grandpa, you'd want an electric scooter that can be brought along even if he goes from one state to another.

There are electric scooter models that are foldable and can fit into a car's trunk easily, so this is the make you might be interested in.

Do you want a scooter with two wheels, three wheels, or four wheels? The additional wheels provide extra support for the rider.

Four wheelers provide maximum stability.

However, do be aware that the more wheels your electric scooter has, the heavier and bulkier it will become. Surely you'd want to buy something that is very safe for your grandpa's use.

Of course, when you're buying an electric scooter, you have to check reviews on it first. If consumer reports showed that it is prone to damage, common sense will tell you to look for another one.

Electronic scooters are not cheap, so you have to make sure that you get the best value for your money.

Chapter 28

4wd Mobility Scooters Keep You Going

Mobility scooters can offer a lot of convenience to individuals that are injured or obese, and need help when it comes to getting from one place to another.

Whether a person is trying to reduce the stress and strain that they put on the bones of their body in order to reduce the risk of an injury, or the individual is simply too frail to get from place to place as quickly as they need to or would like to be able to, mobility scooters can provide a welcome relief to these individuals in that they are then able to accomplish their specific individualized goals when it comes to moving around or from one place to another.

However, these people also want to be able to rely on the safety and reliability of these scooters.

This is essential, since otherwise the individual is not being helped any more than they would be without the scooter. To invest in an item built to move one around, and then not be able to move around in it from time to time would easily be considered by most people to be a waste of money.

This is why many people should look at the specifics of their mobility scooters before they purchase them.

There are many things that can make one type of mobility scooter better than another type of mobility scooter simply because the difference between the two can enable one to be relied on more often than the other one would be.

Prices and characterizations of each mobility scooter need to be considered carefully by consumers in order to ensure that

they are making the right decision when it comes to their
investment in mobility scooters.
The winter time is not only a time in which people are more
likely to get hurt on account of the weather conditions,
but it is also a time in which individuals need to be able to
rely on their mobility scooters outside.
Because of this, many companies have begun to offer 4wd mobility
scooters.
These work in similar ways to 4 wheel drive vehicles.
4wd mobility scooters allow the individual to have more
control over their movements, even on slick or slippery services.
Where less effective mobility scooters may become stuck,
mobility scooters with 4wd are able to get through the difficult
elemental effects of the weather and keep the individual safe
and secure while they are transported from one area to another.
While they are often more expensive, they also offer more
by way of convenience and effective capabilities.
Some people will need to be careful, though.
If a person is living in Arizona, they will probably not need
to purchase a 4wd mobility scooter simply because they are
not exposed to the need for such an item.
Rather, this type of purchase needs to be thought about
carefully, logically and rationally by the consumer prior to
their commitment in purchasing a 4wd mobility scooter
from a manufacturer or other retail outlet, Penny saver ad
or another individual that is parting with their 4wd mobility
scooters.

Chapter 29

The Benefits Of 4 Wheel Mobility Scooters

In stores, we will often come across experiences wherein we observe an individual that is sitting down in a scooter and going about their shopping process.

Sometimes there is a basket attached to the scooter and other times there are not.

We will see them move up and down the aisles, and for the safety of themselves and others they will often beep when they are backing up in order to alert others.

The 4 wheel mobility scooters enable a person to ride along on the scooter much in the manner or a small and personalized car.

The four wheels provide a comfortable situation for the individual to be in, and they easily allow the person to go backwards, forwards, left and right.

This is very beneficial for individuals that are hurt, and still need to go grocery shopping.

For example, if a person breaks one or both of their legs, this will have no effect on their eating schedule.

Even while their legs heal, they will likely still need to eat, play and work.

Having an injury should not prevent a person from performing any of these processes.

The application of a 4 wheel mobility scooter will enable the individual to focus on just these necessary things.

There are different types of scooters that exist on the market today, and 4 wheel mobility scooters were some of the first ones that were produced and put on the market for individuals to invest in when it comes to personalized transportation and assistance.

Not only are they reliable and durable, but they have been around long enough for the manufacturers to understand what is and is not helpful in designing these items. There are more places than individuals may know exist when it comes to outlets for purchasing these types of mobility scooters. Some of us may have observed the commercials on television late at night talking about these mobility scooters, but we are not just limited to purchasing these devices from late night infomercials.

The truth is that there are a number of companies that make these available new to individuals, but there are even more places from which a person can purchase a used mobility scooter with 4 wheels, including from a newspaper's classified ads section, an online auction site or item forum, or from an online store that is selling 4 wheel mobility scooters. The reasons for individuals wanting to purchase these items vary, but for the most part they are purchased by individuals that are caused pain when they are on their feet for a long period of time.

For example, individuals that have any broken bones in their body from the waist down and are trying to heal can benefit. So, too, can individuals that are considered to be overweight, since in some situations this can cause stress and strain on the body, doing more harm than good when it comes to walking around, grocery shopping, for example.

The advantages that this type of device can provide to the individual can vary from person to person, but there are many advantages to discover.

Chapter 30

What Type Of Electric Scooter Is Best For You?

This is a rather subjective issue, but if you're looking for an electric scooter that would be best for your particular situation, then you should consider several factors first before you make a decision.

There are many kinds and makes of electric scooters in the market, so choosing the best one can be a bit confusing.

This article hopes to give you the basic things you need to look for when it comes to buying an electric scooter.

First, find out how much and how often you are going to use it. If you're just getting an electric scooter for emergency use, in case your car breaks down or you need a quick run to the nearby convenience store, then you're better off with the most basic electric scooter model.

You can buy one for as low as $500.

However, if you're buying an electric scooter for everyday use, that is, for somebody who is handicapped or a senior citizen, you might want to invest in the higher models. In fact, the more stable the unit is, the better.

In this case, a four-wheeled electric scooter is your best choice.

There are other types of electric scooters out there.

You can have something that has just two wheels, while you can also own one that has three wheels.

Of course, the four wheeler is the most stable and should be the one you're getting for your parents or, if you want, for your kid.

It would also be best to buy an electric scooter that won't take up so much space in your garage.

The bulky scooters are not as big as cars, but they occupy garage space, nonetheless.

If your parking lot is already cramped, you might want to buy an electric scooter that can easily be folded up. If you travel a lot and intend to bring your electric scooter around, you should buy something that can be disassembled.

Just make sure you know how to put it back, of course.

Choosing the right kind of electric scooter can be a pretty daunting task.

But if you know what you need and determined your budget, this should be a pretty easy decision.

Electric scooters are not just functional, they can also be trendy. So, aside from its use, you should also factor in how it looks when you make that purchase.

Chapter 31

Electric Mobility Scooters And What To Look For

Electric mobility scooters are designed to assist those who
have physical conditions that make walking difficult enjoy
the sense of independence and freedom that comes from mobility.
When selecting the appropriate make and model of
an electric scooter the individual rider's overall physical
condition and personal preferences need to be considered in
relation to the basic construction of the scooter.
The basic construction should combine a backrest, seat and
foot support to provide a comfortable and stable seating base.
This enables riders to expend their energy on the
essential activities, such as operating the vehicle and
accomplishing tasks from within the mobility scooter rather
than wasting effort trying to maintain a comfortable, upright
position.
The seat unit should have an anatomically contoured seat
 base and backrest and be wide enough to accommodate
outdoor clothing if necessary.
However, it should not be so wide that the user is forced to sit
asymmetrically to feel properly supported.
 If the seat is too narrow it will become uncomfortable and
increase the risk of pressure sores.
Try to choose an electric mobility scooter that has a seat and
backrest which can be adjusted to meet individual comfort levels.
Additionally, a seat with fold up armrests adds to the
comfort of the rider, make transferring on and off the seat

easier and will reduce the amount of physical strain on the upper body. A stable seating posture is essential in order to manage the vehicle's controls which are located on the tiller, or steering column and handlebars. The tiller is the control and steering mechanism for the mobility scooter and has the controls to drive the scooter forward or in reverse, as well as steering the front wheels. Some tillers feature height and angle adjustability to ensure that the rider can comfortably reach the tiller and therefore has maximum control over the scooter.

A console, centrally located on the tiller, has the supplementary controls for lights, indicators, horn and to power the unit on and off. Two hands are typically required to manage the tiller steering component of an electric mobility scooter.

Some models can be controlled by only one hand if the model is equipped with one level for acceleration that switches for forward and reverse mode, however operating supplementary controls at the same time as steering can be difficult.

If the intended rider is interested in an electric mobility scooter that will travel as well as provide travel you will want to investigate transportable electric mobility scooters. Transportable mobility scooters can be dismantled for transport and storage.

On larger scooters or those intended for rugged outdoor use, you may want to check the weight of the largest individual piece in order to be properly prepared to disassemble as individual components can still be quite heavy.

Although a convenient feature, when you consider transporting a mobility scooter you will have to keep in mind that transporting the scooter will require it to be broken down before the next destination, assembled upon arrival, disassembled upon return and once again assembled for use at home.

This may not seem very convenient, but when it comes to being able to join family and friends on a special outing or having to choose to not participate due to physical limitations, the break down and set up of the mobility scooter is a more than worthwhile small chore in comparison to the benefits it brings to the rider and their ability to interact independently with family and friends.

Chapter 32

Exploring Bruno Mobility Scooters

When it comes to the world of mobility scooters, there are a fair number of manufacturers that are considered to be reliable, durable and dependable.

These more elite brands are easily relied on by the individual because they have been able to prove their worth over the period of time that they have been in existence and established. Bruno mobility scooters are some of the most reliable scooters that have been available for purchase on the open market and they are designed for particular reasons and purposes.

Like almost all mobility scooters, they are intended to be used for individuals that would need assistance moving around. Sometimes this is caused when a person suffers an injury. For example, if an individual has broken both of their feet in an accident, they will need something like a Bruno mobility scooter simply because they will not be able to put any pressure on their feet while they are healing.

Instead, they will need to be transported.

Wheelchairs are an option, but for individuals waiting for the bones in their feet to heal, this may not be a good loan term solution to the problem.

Bruno mobility scooters will allow the individual to be easily transported to and from destinations, but at the same time they will be comfortable and able to relax.

The last thing anyone needs is more stress and strain put on them,

especially when it comes to individuals that are attempting
to heal.

By ensuring that the individual is kept in a comfortable and
strain-free position, they are able to focus more on healing
and stay in more positive spirits, instead of sinking into a
possible depression as a result of not being able to move
around as easily as they once were able to do.

Another example of individuals that would be able to benefit
from the use of Bruno mobility scooters would be those who are
overweight. Being overweight can put a lot of stress and
strain on the body when it is being moved around.

Rather than put stress and strain on the bones, effectively
Increasing the odds of injury or accident, it can be easier and
More convenient for the individuals to use Bruno mobility
Scooters until such a time that the individual is able to reduce
their weight.

Since this can sometimes be a lengthy process, many
people would benefit in the meantime from utilizing the
Bruno mobility scooters that are available for purchase, both
in new and used conditions.

By being able to rely on a device that will allow the individual
to move about easily and conveniently, it is more likely that
these individuals would open themselves up to new experiences
since they no longer have to worry about putting their body in a
potentially dangerous position.

Despite the fact that it seems like the person would be less active,
the truth is that be finding something to benefit them when it
comes to being able to go out and do things, they will actually
be increasing their activity levels.

Chapter 33

The Perks Of An Electric Motor Scooter

Before electric motor scooters were invented, handicapped people had no choice but to contend with a limited mobile life.

Sure, a wheelchair can get them from one point of the house to another, but it doesn't have the ability to travel long distances.

On the contrary, an electric motor scooter can bring them from the house to the grocery store and back effortlessly, so they don't feel cooped up and useless.

The key thrust of electric motor scooter sales is independence.

Because it allows the handicapped and the elderly to move about without having to ask help from anyone, it boosts their self esteem.

No longer will they have to worry about bothering anyone about performing daily mundane tasks and the better they start feeling about themselves.

While there are also gas powered scooters, electric motor scooters are more convenient to use.

This is because you no longer need to go to the gas station to fill up.

All you need to do is plug the electric motor scooter into an electrical outlet and wait a couple of hours for it recharge fully.

After which, you can start enjoying another trip around the

neighbourhood again. Electric motor scooters also come in portable and foldable versions.
 If you travel around a lot, you can simply fold up
or disassemble your electric motor scooter and the plane won't even scold you for it.
Electric scooters can go as light as 22 pounds.
The average price of electric motor scooters is $800, but you can already own one for as low as $580.
This is still pretty expensive, though, but once the demand starts to catch on, the price of electric motor scooters is
 expected to go down.
Soon, everyone will be wanting an electric motor scooter of their own.
Of course, before you buy an electric motor scooter, be sure that that particular model is really what you need.
There are different versions of electric scooters so it would be best to obtain information from the Internet first before you sign that receipt.
Electric scooters are practical, yes, but if you find
no use for it in your personal life and would just like to get with the fad, then you better rethink your decision.

Chapter 34

Before You Buy An Electric Scooter, Read Reviews

As a consumer, it is your personal responsibility to ensure that everything you spend on delivers the value you expect for its price.

This is the same principle you should practice when it comes to buying electric scooters.

That is, before you make any decisions and sign that receipt, you should first see what the reviews are saying about that particular model.

There aren't many electronic scooters showcased at physical motor and vehicles stores, so you won't be able to scrutinize everything.

However, you can make your initial assessments based on the reviews you find on the Internet.

While it is true that not all reviews are genuine, as review fabrication is one of the tactics some marketers use, exposing yourself to different review sites will help give you a general idea about a certain product.

If you don't want to rely on just any kind of review, you can always check with Consumer Reports or Best Buy for up to date and well researched assessments of various products, including electric scooters.

These sources are reliable because they truly test the products they review.

So are sure to be getting just the right kind of information.

What should you look for in an electric scooter review?

First, when the review and testing was done.

Second, who did it and how.

Third, his observations regarding the electric scooter's manueverability, stability, features, safety, price, and the manufacturer's customer service offerings.

Fourth, if the scooter is eligible for upgrades and add-ons. Just because an electric scooter looks good on the outside, doesn't mean it's good to go.

What is important in an electric scooter is that it can serve its purpose well and won't give you any headaches in the future. Reviews are very important in helping you make the right choice. Take advantage of them.

Chapter 35

Repairing Your Electric Scooter

Like any other piece of equipment, your electric scooter is also subject to potential wear. Just because it's pretty compact and doesn't use gas to run does not mean that it is forever spared from possible breakdowns.

So, if your electric scooter unit bogs down, where can you take it? Are there any electric scooter repair shops around? Fortunately for you, because an electric scooter operates on a simple and commonplace electric mechanism, you can have it repaired at a local electronics or motorcycle shops.

Some shops that have absolutely no experience with electric scooters might get intimidated and turn you down, but it's really not complicated to redo at all.

If going to neighbourhood repair shops is not an option for you, you can contact the dealer who sold you the scooter and ask where you can have it fixed.

More likely, the dealer will also have people who know how to repair these kinds of vehicles, so you can just as well consider it a one-stop shop.

Also, check if your unit is still covered by the warranty so you can have it repaired for free.

It will probably take just a few days to repair your scooter. For minor damage, you might even only need to wait a few hours to get it back up and running again.

Overall, you shouldn't expect your electric scooter to be free of hassles forever.

Because it also gets tired from constant use, it will expectedly give out at some point.

But, if you also do not use your electric scooter often, the under-use could also contribute to the damage.

If you don't plan on using it regularly, make sure it is properly stored and placed away from moisture.

You paid quite a price for your electric scooter.

And while you don't wear it down with constant use, the least you can do it maintain it well.

Chapter 36

The Different Uses Of Electric Scooters

Electric scooters are not just for the elderly and the handicapped. Anybody who'd want greater convenience in life, or even just a new hobby to tinker with can benefit from owning an electric scooter.

The use of the electric scooter is not confined to simply transporting a person from one place to another. If you're creative, you can find a lot of different ways to enjoy your scooter ride.

Here are some possible uses for your electric scooter:

1) They are perfect to use for carrying loads the car cannot in emergency situations.

For instance, if you need to take a certain equipment to the repair shop and the car is not around, you will have no problem doing so if you have an electric scooter.

In addition, you won't even have to think about contributing pollutants to the atmosphere.

2) If you need to make a short trip to the neighbourhood grocery, your electric scooter will come in handy. Some models have carrying baskets in front or compartments beneath to place your purchases in, but some users have been seen comfortably hanging their bags on the handlebars.

3) While electric scooters may not be used on rough terrain, you can still bring them along when you go camping to enjoy on fairly flat surfaces. There are certain e-scooter models that you can easily pack and fold for trips like these. Your kids will surely appreciate you bringing it along.

4) You can maneuver through heavy traffic and never be late for work or a meeting ever again. Unless, of course, you really meant to be.

5) If you're bored, you can cruise around town on your electric scooter. It could be a great place to spend alone time and do some thinking.

These are just a few of the many things you can do with an electric scooter, even if you are not mobility impaired. With a little creativity and true recognition of the machine's functionality, you will be able to maximize the use of your electric scooter. After all, you paid for it. You might as well get maximum value for your money.

Chapter 37

Finding Electric Scooters For Sale

The popularity of electric scooters is fast rising nowadays, what with the growing need for a more practical vehicle to manoeuvre through heavy traffic and the continuing increase in gas and fuel prices.

Having said this, if you're looking to find electric scooters for sale, you won't have trouble finding where they are.

You will see electric scooters for sale all over the Internet. What you need to do is just type 'electric scooters for sale' on the search engine of your choice and you will be faced with literally hundreds of online stores offering all kinds and makes of electric scooters.

You can choose from a two-wheel drive, a three-wheel drive, or a four-wheel drive. In short, everything you need on electric scooters can be found on the Internet.

You can also see electric scooters for sale on local motorcycle shops.

Because electric scooters are fast becoming the vehicle of choice for many, finding several of these babies on motor shops will not be a problem.

However, you might not find all models in one store.

Your best option, if this is the case, is to contact the manufacturer directly ask for a catalogue of their products.

Another great source of electric scooters on sale are forums. Here, not only will you be able to buy all sorts of electric scooters, but you might also chance upon customized versions, as well as used ones.

Since electric scooters retail for around $700, you might find something as low as $350 at the forums.

It's going to be already used, of course, so just make sure that you know all the details about the unit before you make a deal.

The popularity of electric scooters might entice you to buy the first thing you see on the market just so you can say that you own one.

However, consider purchasing an electric scooter for its function and purpose.

An electric scooter is not just something you can use to cruise around the block with.

You can actually use it to go to work. For some models, they can even go as fast as ten miles per hour, so you're also not lacking in the speed department.

To reiterate, an electric scooter is not merely a stylish piece of equipment.

If you know how to use it, you will be able to maximize its full benefits.

Chapter 38

How Can You Benefit From An Electric Scooter?

Almost anybody can benefit from owning an electric scooter. Aside from the convenience of just plugging the unit to an electrical outlet to make it work, you no longer need to spend so much on gas, especially at a time that world oil prices are continuing to skyrocket.

Scooters are very easy to use. Apart from being relatively cheap compared to cars, they also get you to your destination faster.

It's small size will enable any rider to maneuver through even the heaviest of traffic jams.

And with its varying speed selections, thrill seekers see it as a vehicle of choice.

While electric scooters are still expensive in the long run, as they will still eat up your electricity consumption, it affords the owner convenience.

And for most people, this convenience is worth the electric bill increase.

Because electric scooters and any other type of scooter for that matter are also not contrived, people who love the open will get a kick out of it.

It will not protect you from the rain, however, but some people do find romance in bathing in the rain while rushing through the streets on a scooter.

But, of course, that's very subjective.

Even the elderly and the handicapped can benefit from owning an electric scooter.

If they found it difficult to get from one place to another before, they can do so easily if they are on an electric scooter.

It's not advisable to use an electric scooter on long trips, though, but if you just want to get to the nearby park or the local grocery store, you won't have any trouble.

Another benefit of electric scooters is that they are portable.

So even if you travel far, you can still bring it along.

Some scooters are foldable so they're very convenient to pack.

This mobile lifestyle is a must have for senior citizens and the handicapped, and, basically, just about anyone who wants to get around town without having to walk.

And with the technology covering electric scooters continuing to advance, it won't be a surprise if we will see better and a lot cheaper versions as the demand rises in the coming years.

Scooters are fun to use.

And with an electric scooter, no longer will you need to fuss over gas prices.

Wherever there is an outlet, you can easily recharge and be on the go again.

Chapter 39

Finding The Best Electric Scooters Around

Thanks to the Internet, finding the right kind of electric scooter to suit your needs has been simplified by just a few clicks of the mouse.

No longer will you need to go from store to store just to come upon the perfect model.

All you need to do is type in what you need and outcome hundreds of sites offering it.

But finding what scooter is for you is not solved by simply logging on to the net.

Since there are many scooter models that more or less meet your expectations, you will still be facing a choice in the end. This is where reviews come in.

If you're eyeing a particular brand and version, be sure to check out what past and present owners and users have to say about the product before deciding to buy it.

This is the practice that is recommended with any other kind of purchase, so the same should be applied when you're trying to find the scooter of your dreams (and budget).

It's not difficult to search the Net for electric scooters.

The challenge lies in the choosing and in the confirming of The veracity of the reviews written about it.

Don't just settle at one site to get all the information you need about your electric scooter.

Try to look up at least five sites and compare their opinions
and descriptions to be sure.

After all, you'll be spending good money on this machine, so
you might as well be very vigilant at the onset.

There are electric scooters for different sizes and for different
functions.

If you're the outdoorsy type, you will find that a four wheel
electric scooter works best with nature trips and if you're just
looking to cruise around the neighbourhood, the 22 pound
electric scooters will suffice.

In short, how you can successfully find the perfect electric
scooter depends on why you want to buy one and what your
budget dictates.

But if you've found the perfect model but hesitate because
it's way beyond your budget, you can again search the
Internet for used versions of the same model and
see if you can get it at half the price.

Happy hunting!

Chapter 40

Travel Light With Your Electric Powered Scooter or Chair

Scooters are low maintenance vehicles. You don't have to
worry about space in the garage if you own a scooter, and
never again will you have to fuss over heavy traffic.
Indeed, scooters can manoeuvre through the tightest of jams
and take you to anyplace you want without fear of getting
stuck and becoming extremely late somewhere.
To add, you can also kiss elusive car parking slots goodbye.
As if scooters are still not great machines, some innovative
minds have come up with electric powered scooters.
The product is relatively new so not everyone might already
know about it.
In fact, we rarely see electric powered scooters cruising the streets.
But that does not discount the fact that they are very practical
to use, especially at a time oil and gas prices are showing no
signs of backing down.
An electric powered scooter, as its name suggests, is run
using electricity.
The unit is hooked up to an outlet, charged and then used.
If the battery shows signs of weakening, you will need to
recharge so it doesn't conk out on you in the middle of nowhere.
Some critics have also panned the idea of an electric powered
scooter because they say it is a burden on one's electricity
bill.
However, its fans argue that it is a great solution to the

world's dependence on oil and gas, which are fast becoming
scarce.
Electric powered scooters come in various sizes and designs.
Like the regular scooters, they also can run in different
speeds.
So if you want to just cruise around suburbia, you
have your electric powered scooter to assure you that your
feet won't get tired.
For now, electric powered scooters are still a little expensive.
But when the product catches on and the demand increases,
it will become more accessible to many people.
A lot of us always complain about always being late to somewhere
because of traffic.
Now, you can go from one place to another in just a short time.
The best thing is, you won't even have to burn fuel anymore,
so you're also doing the environment a favor.

Chapter 41

Appreciating Electric Motorized Scooters

Everybody is into convenience these days. For instance, electric motorized scooters, which have originally been designed for people with very limited mobile capacities, have found their way into the hands of ordinary people who just want to get away from the hassle of owning cars.

While we're not saying that car ownership is a lot of trouble, the fact that electric scooters are offering a quicker alternative to get a certain destination is the reason why its popularity is fast rising.

And with the worsening of traffic conditions, it won't be a surprise if every household has at least one electric motorized scooter in its garage.

An electric motorized scooter, as its name suggests, is run using electricity.

The unit is hooked up to an outlet, charged and then used. If the battery shows signs of weakening, you will need to recharge so it doesn't conk out on you in the middle of nowhere.

Some critics have even panned the idea of an electric scooter because they say it is a burden on one's electricity bill. However, its fans argue that it is a great solution to the world's dependence on oil and gas, which are fast becoming scarce.

The main goal of an electric motorized scooter is to provide convenience.
Because traffic can be such a headache, the size
of scooters allows its riders to just breeze through and get to their destinations even faster than taking a car or a cab on a normal day.
And because scooters have varying speeds, thrill
seekers (and people who are always on the go) will benefit greatly from this piece of equipment.
In short, electric motorized scooters are not just for those who have trouble moving around. They can also be a great advantage to those who just want to enjoy their surroundings without being delayed by traffic and other conditions.

Chapter 42

How To Choose Your Electric Scooter Or Bike

Scooters are probably one of the most convenient and easy to use vehicles around. Unlike a car, you don't really have to go through driving school to be able to handle a scooter safely. Sometimes, all you even have to have is the knowledge on how to ride an ordinary bike and you're good to go.

If you're planning on doing tricks with your electric scooter, however, you will have to go through another kind of training, of course.

What is it about scooters that appeals to us? Perhaps it is fact that scooters are so small that they can outmanoeuvre any car at any place.

Because we live at a time where traffic jams are commonplace, owning a scooter or a bike is one of the most practical decisions we can have.

How do we choose an electric scooter or bike? Given the fact that there are several types of electric scooters, choosing the right one to suit our needs can be a challenge.

For instance, do you want an electric scooter or bike that can be disassembled for easy storage? Are you planning to bring this scooter around with you when you travel? There are electric scooter or bike models that can be as light as 22 pounds, so even if you are intending to board a plane it won't be a nuisance.

You can also choose between a two wheeler, three wheeler, and four wheeler.

Naturally, the four wheeler models are the heaviest and bulkiest, but if safety is your concern, or if you're buying

an electric scooter or bike for someone who is handicapped,
you should choose on a four-wheel version.

Speed limits on electric scooters or bikes are lower than the
regular gas powered scooters, but they are fast nonetheless.
Just because they run on electricity doesn't mean they're of
the wimpy sort.

Electric scooters and bikes are not just toys to make you look cute.
They are actually very functional.

The average price of an electric scooter or bike is $800,
but you can own one for as low as $580.

Now that you know the basics about electric scooters or
bikes, it is hoped that you will make a better decision with
your purchase.

Chapter 43

Benefits Of 3 Wheel Mobility Scooters

One of the most common types of mobility scooters are those that were manufactured and produced with four wheels.
They are able to go forwards, backwards and of course left and right.
For quite a while they were considered to be very useful and helpful, and many people appreciated the efficiency and convenience that devices like them offered to the individuals that needed the assistance.
However, over time, as technology advanced, individuals began to start expecting more of all their technologically backed items, including mobility scooters.
And so, as companies began to make more changes on their mobility scooters, in order to make them more appealing to consumers, eventually some companies came up with the idea o design mobility scooters that would be able to function with fewer wheels, and offer even more to the individual by way of efficiency, convenience and style.
This is part of what makes them so appealing and attractive to consumers and individuals that are thinking about purchasing such items, if they find that they have begun to need something to help them move around from one place to another.
Sometimes this happens when a person succumbs to an injury, and in other instances these devices are used by

individuals that would otherwise feel pain when moving about at such a steady pace or for such a lengthy period of time.

Most people would not think so, but mobility scooters are not like an individual's car. They want items and devices that will help them to feel good about themselves.

They want items that will look nice and sharp 3 wheel mobility scooters offer not only cutting edge technology and convenience, but they are also able to offer a new look to individuals that are considering investing in such items.

They are designed to look more streamlined and aerodynamic, not unlike a car.

The rounded edges and sturdy design help to make 3 wheel mobility scooters popular, but this is not what clenches it for these types of scooters.

Rather, it is the different things that an individual can do with the 3 wheel mobility scooters that help to put them ahead when it comes to the benefits and advantages that come with the scooter.

Not limited to rough turns or three point turns, the one singular wheel in the front of three wheel mobility scooters allows the individual to move around in a much more fluid motion.

People no longer need to go forward, then back, and then forward again in order to complete a sharp turn.

Instead, the new more subtle look of the scooter and the unassuming design help the individual in charge of the 3 wheel mobility scooter to move in a more simple and steady form.

This makes these types of mobility scooters more appealing to consumers because they offer efficiency, and extended convenience in addition to style and sleek designs which can help to make a person feel better about admitting that they may need help moving around from time to time.

No one likes to feel helpless, and a mobility scooter such as this can add an exciting edge to the event.

Chapter 44

The Conquest Wheelchair Motorcycle

While the automobile is often times used as a metaphor for freedom, there are no vehicles that offer the total freedom of a motorcycle.

For those who are physically disabled below the waist and who harbor a love for exploring the open road in something more liberating than a car or van, that freedom is attainable once again through our wheelchair accessible motorcycle.

Combining the highest-quality materials, a powerful engine and an innovative design, The Conquest wheelchair motorcycle is made especially for those who can no longer ride a standard motorcycle, but who are not ready to give up the exhilaration of riding a motorbike, and a big one at that.

The three-wheel Conquest Wheelchair Motorcycle, by Mobility Conquest, is uniquely designed to accommodate any physically disabled rider.

With the help of a rearward ramp, riders can mount their wheelchairs onto the driving platform.

Within 7.6 seconds, you can experience the thrills of freedom and adventure on the open road!

The Conquest wheelchair motorcycle has an 1170 CC engine that can keep up with — and probably outrun quite a bit of the competition.

This three-wheel motorcycle trike can hit 60 mph within 7.6 seconds of leaving the line. The top speed is a blazing 105 mph, too fast for the highways, but certainly enough to guarantee that you will never run short of power when it's needed.

The wheelchair motorcycle's stylish design makes it something unique on the road.

The Conquest doesn't mean riding alone.

This handicap accessible motorcycle can take passengers along for the ride and high-end suspension at both ends of the motorbike means that handling and control aren't compromised by extra weight.

The chassis offers remarkable stability without losing the precise manoeuvrability for which motorcycles are known, and loved.

The driver mounts the wheelchair accessible motorcycle via an automatic rearward ramp.

The trike accommodates both the driver and their wheelchair by a secure locking mechanism with a push-button release to ensure a stable driving platform.

All our handicap accessible trikes come with a reverse gear for ease of manoeuvrability and parking.

The push button shift controls makes accelerating through the motorbike's six gears a breeze.

The Conquest makes the open road accessible to anyone who craves the thrill of being on a motorcycle.

Chapter 45

The Best Electric Scooter Brands

There are many electric scooter brands out there, but not all are as reliable or positively reviewed as the ones we will be mentioning here. In fact, most people have this misconception that any electric scooter is just as good as another.

This is where we are wrong.

How the machine is made and what features it carries should be the basis for judging if an electric scooter is worth your money or not.

Oh, yes Electric scooters are not just mobile thingies you plug in order to run.

Like their gas powered counterparts, they have features.

What are the best electric scooter brands in the market today? Here are five of them, in no particular order.

1) The Pride Mobility Sundancer

It's one of the best three wheel electric scooters around because of its easy manoeuvrability despite the fact that it's a little larger than usual.

2) Drive's Phantom 3-Wheel Scooter

Though it has a small design, it is not lacking in power. It has a swivel seats that has several locking position and an adjustable armrest for greater transferring convenience. Aside from being very easy to drive around, it also can be folded down and fit into any car trunk.

3) Shoprider Mobility's Sunrunner 4
It weighs 300 pounds but all of that is offset by its many features, which include electromagnetic brakes, a 50 inch turning radius, headlights, a front basket and a deluxe captain's seat.

4) Golden Technologies 4-Wheel Companion
The best feature of this wonderful vehicle is that it can automatically shut down when not in use, thus, saving power.

5) The Pride Hurricane PMV
This is the best unit for those who want speed, too. It can run for as fast as 9 miles per hour despite weighing 400 pounds! People with problems with mobility will surely benefit from owning an electric scooter. They are designed with their users' safety and convenience in mind. However, while you might be compelled to think that you can't go wrong with any electric scooter, heed the above advice to get the best the market has to offer.

Chapter 46

Choosing A Power Chairs

Go Chair

The first travel chair that combines super portability, manoeuvrability and style at a low, low cost. The Go-Chair has an easy to remove battery pack, a compact lightweight frame and conveniently disassembles into four manageable pieces to fit into the boot of most vehicles.

Maximum speed 5.6km/h, length 68.5cm, width 48cm, range up to 16km, component weights front section 10kg, rear section 16kg, seat 11kg, batteries 9kg. Weight capacity 113kg

Jazzy Select

The highly manoeuvrable Jazzy SelectTM delivers the advantages of in-line motor technology for enhanced efficiency, torque, range, and performance. Plus, it s loaded with performance and convenience features, like standard Active-Trac Suspension, that make it as easy to enjoy as it is to use.

Jazzy Select 14XL

The Jazzy SelectTM 14 Series delivers the advantages of patented mid-wheel drive for maneuvering in tight, compact spaces. Both the Jazzy Select 14 and Jazzy Select 14 XL are loaded with performance and convenience features like a powerful 60 amp PG VR2 controller, larger batteries for greater per-charge range, and on-board battery charger.

The Rascal

This brand has more than 10 different models. It is suitable for indoor and outdoor use.

The heavy duty models suit most users, sturdy and powerful enough to accommodate up to lbs. 550

To find more information visit their website: http://www.rascal.com

End Note

This book was written with the aim to help inform people who by some misfortune find themselves in need of a Mobility Devise, be it a wheel chair or a Mobility scooter.
 I endeavoured to add as many details as possible.
There are a great number of Mobility Devises; I chose to concentrate on Electric Scooters and Chairs, as they seem to be the ones most used by handicapped people, the elderly and children.
These devises make everyday living a lot easier.
I also tried to include information related to **Motorcycle** lovers, regardless of the fact that motorcycles are a contributing factor to a person needing a Mobility Devise, but then so are motor vehicles.
In case you would like more information or would like to contact me visit; http://www.electricmobilitychairs.com

Mema Manna

ABOUT THE AUTHOR

Mema Manna is an author, teacher, mother and grandmother. After retiring from a teaching career she discovered the exciting world of online business and all the opportunities that running an Internet business can bring.

She wrote a number of books related to her teaching while working for "Victoria University of Technology" in Melbourne, Australia.

Her philosophy is that life doesn't stop at retirement; whatever your age, there are opportunities before your eyes all the time; all you have to do is open your eyes and mind to them.

She is, and has been married for 38 plus years, has 2 lovely sons and 1 beautiful granddaughter. Life is wonderful and interesting, never a dull moment that is for sure.

So here begins another journey in her life.

www.ingramcontent.com/pod-product-compliance
Lightning Source LLC
Chambersburg PA
CBHW081839280526
45789CB00007B/2504